What the Bible says about Healing and Prosperity

Ed Harding

New Wine Press

New Wine Ministries
PO Box 17
Chichester
West Sussex
United Kingdom
PO19 2AW

Copyright © 2011 Edward Harding

All rights reserved. No part of this publication may be reproduced, stored in a retrieval system, or transmitted in any form or by any means, electronic, mechanical, photocopying or otherwise, without the prior written consent of the publisher. Short extracts may be used for review purposes.

Scripture quotations are taken from the King James Bible, Crown Copyright unless stated as follows:
   NKJV – New King James Version. Copyright © 1982 by Thomas Nelson Inc. Nashville, USA. Used by permission.
   NIV – The Holy Bible New International Version. Copyright © 1973, 1978, 1984, 2011 by Biblica Inc. Used by permission. All rights reserved worldwide.

ISBN 978-1-905991-71-6

Text design and typesetting by **documen**, www.documen.co.uk
Cover design by Stephen Coleman
Printed in Malta

Contents

	About the Author	4
	Introduction	5
Chapter 1	Genesis and the Fall	7
Chapter 2	The Three Sources of Sickness	12
Chapter 3	The Effects of the Curse	17
Chapter 4	Christ our Redeemer	19
Chapter 5	Physical or Spiritual?	22
Chapter 6	Biblical Methods of Healing	25
Chapter 7	Blockages to Healing	28
Chapter 8	What to do if You're Sick	30
Chapter 9	Finally... never give up	35
Chapter 10	For Me to Live is Christ, to Die is Gain	37
Chapter 11	What is Prosperity?	40

About the Author

Ed Harding believes passionately in divine healing and the full restoration of all the gifts and ministries God wants in the Body of Christ. He has been taking ministry teams overseas for a number of years, especially to India, to preach the Gospel with signs following.

Ed has seen a number of spectacular miracles with many people healed and delivered from demonic oppression, and he has also seen many people who have not been healed. He wants to extend the teaching ministry through books such as this to see God's people come into full understanding and blessing.

Since this teaching was first published many people have been saved and healed, including a healing revival in India. May this be true for you, whatever your need is. God really does have the answer.

Introduction

Healing is probably the most controversial and contentious issue which Christians face in the Church today. You may well know someone who says they have been healed by God's supernatural power. You will also, most likely, know of those with good Christian character who have not recovered despite much prayer and intercession on their behalf. At one extreme there are those who believe and teach that everyone should be healed if only they learned how to appropriate the scriptures and had enough faith. At the other extreme there are those who believe that God does not intervene to heal supernaturally today, and to teach that He does raises false hopes. Indeed, worse than that, they say it is a cruel deception which leaves the victim in unreality and quite unprepared for death.

The shock then affects the family. What if they had prayed more? Did they have too little faith? Why did God ignore their prayers? What about all those promises in the Bible? If you then consider all the apparent unjust suffering of, for example, children with terminal illnesses, where is God in it all? Where is His love and compassion?

In this short book we will try to address some of these issues to see precisely what Scripture teaches, both for the believer and the unbeliever.

As a personal introduction I have, over some 40 years as a Christian, been healed by God of conditions for which I was receiving specialist medical treatment, seen God do some spectacular miracles, and also witnessed the death of good, solid Christian friends.

Should everybody expect to be healed in all circumstances or is healing conditional? If so what are the conditions? Or did it all cease with the apostles?

But before we address such questions we have to go right back to the beginning. We need to know where sickness comes from. As is so often the case, the key lies in Genesis.

CHAPTER 1

Genesis and the Fall

Just as you will never understand your salvation properly until you understand the Fall of Man, equally I believe you need to see what precisely happened at that time when the whole human race fell under God's judgement, to understand sickness, the effects of sin and how God made provision for Adam and mankind.

In Genesis 2:17 Adam is forbidden to eat of the tree of the knowledge of good and evil *"for when you eat of it you will surely die"* (NIV). Literally it translates 'dying you shall die'. Up to that point Adam had eternal life, a perfect disease-free body created for eternity, and had he not sinned would still be here now! Incidentally that's why God will create a new heaven **and** a new earth, because it's the perfect environment for man and is part of the divine plan of restoration of all things. Those who think only heaven is our final destination are in for a most wonderful surprise!

The effects of the Fall of Man were devastating:

To the serpent God said *"**Cursed** are you above all the livestock."*

(Genesis 3:14)

To the woman God said *"I will greatly increase your **pains** in childbearing; with **pain** you will give birth to children."*

(Genesis 3:16)

> To Adam God said *"**Cursed** is the ground because of you; through **painful** toil you will eat of it... By the sweat of your brow you will eat your food until you return to the ground."*
>
> (Genesis 3:17,19 NIV)

Hence the whole human race came under God's judgement, with toil, sweat, tears and finally death. Man had fallen. Worse was to come.

Initially, if you read Genesis 5, you'll see that Adam lived to be 930 years old (verse 5), Seth lived to 912 years (verse 8), Enoch 905 (verse 11), Kenan 910 (verse 14), and so it goes on, naming ages of 895, 962, 365, (Enoch who never died) 969 and 777 years. Then there is a further phase of judgement – God shortens life to 120 years, basically because of sin. Note what God says:

> *"My Spirit will not contend with man for ever: for he is mortal; his days will be a hundred and twenty years."*
>
> (Genesis 6:3)

Why? Verse 11 tells us *"Now the earth was corrupt in God's sight and was full of violence..."* As a consequence, all of mankind was destroyed in a global flood over the whole earth together with all the animals apart from those in the ark. That judgement had a dramatic effect on the world's climate, eradicating huge areas of vegetation, and causing many species of animals to die out.

Although we're perhaps more familiar with God's promise never to flood the earth again, God made another promise:

> *"Never again will I curse the ground because of man, even though every inclination of his heart is evil from childhood."*
>
> (Genesis 8:21)

This expresses His heart. God must judge sin, but He wants to bless.

You may wonder what this has to do with healing, but unless you diagnose the root cause of sickness correctly you won't apply the correct remedy. Sickness was part of the judgement at the Fall. By the time of King David, God had shortened life even more:

> "The length of our days is seventy years – or eighty if we have the strength."
>
> (Psalm 90:10)

In the twenty-first Century the average age span in Western nations has in fact risen to over eighty, largely due to medical technology prolonging life, rather than natural strength as in David's day. Long life is seen as a blessing in the Bible, a short life a curse. That's not just a promise linked to the commandment to honour your father and mother, but the theme runs right through Scripture. Perhaps the clearest expression of God's intention is in Isaiah 65:20 which describes the reign of Christ on earth:

> "Never again will there be in it an infant that lives but a few days, or an old man who does not live out his years; he who dies at a hundred will be thought a mere youth: **he who fails to reach a hundred will be considered accursed.**"

So where is this all leading? It shows that **all** of mankind is still under the curse of a shortened life, the ageing process, decay and finally death. You may wonder why I say that everyone is under the curse of decay, but the answer is actually very simple. You cannot die without a bodily malfunction. It is simply impossible! Whether you are shot in a war or die in your sleep the doctor writing your death certificate has to state a cause of death. Parts of the body stop functioning – that's how you die! The wonderful truth about our new resurrection bodies is, of course, that because believers have everlasting life in their new bodies they don't get sick either. Just as decay and death go together, equally health and everlasting life go together. It is inconceivable that we will be sick in heaven! Paul writes to the Romans in Romans 8:19-24 explaining precisely what I have been describing:

> *"The creation waits in eager expectation for the sons of God to be revealed. For the creation was subjected to frustration, not by its own choice, but by the will of the one who subjected it, in hope, that the creation itself will be liberated from its **bondage to decay** and brought into the glorious freedom of the children of God.*
>
> *We know that the whole creation has been groaning as in the pains of childbirth right up to the present time. Not only so, but we ourselves, who have the firstfruits of the Spirit, groan inwardly as we wait eagerly for our adoption as sons, the **redemption of our bodies.**"*
>
> (NIV)

It is quite clear that we are not going to get our new sickness-free resurrection bodies right now. As Paul writes in verse 25:

"we wait for it patiently."

Because all creation is in bondage to decay, you will grow old, acquire wrinkles, change shape, and become increasingly prone to sickness. The Bible never promises eternal youth. Indeed Proverbs 31:30 on the perfect wife tells us:

"Charm is deceptive, and beauty is fleeting."

We need to lay this foundation from Genesis and understand the Fall. Christians are not divinely immune from sickness, as we shall see later. Nor should you feel any guilt in consulting a doctor if you're sick. You are no worse than the rest of the human race. Of course you should seek God first about your sickness and what treatment to take.

After a ministry trip in Nigeria some years ago I developed flu symptoms. I soldiered on at work. Eventually I saw a doctor who took some blood, but nothing showed up. I carried on, eventually collapsing into bed with a fever. I could scarcely stand up. More blood was taken and analysed. I had falciparum malaria, the most dangerous type, which can kill you in 48 hours. I was duly taken to hospital, arriving with a blood pressure of 60 over zero. Zero means there isn't any to measure! My wife insisted I had immediate treatment or there might not be a patient to treat at all. I was given the corrective treatment and duly recovered. I believe God spared my life and sustained me until I got proper medical treatment. I didn't blame the devil, or claim the automatic right to divine healing. I recognised that my human body is in bondage to decay, and needed corrective medical treatment. Certainly I was healed and even had to sign a government form to say I hadn't died!

Christians have been made to feel guilty for being sick and lacking in faith if they consult a doctor. Some have even denied they were sick at all and died as a result. The sensible Christian will strike the right balance between seeking God, prayer, common sense eating and exercise, and remembering that we are basically still under the curse of the Fall. Later we will cover what it means when Christ became a curse for us and redeemed us.

As we shall now see, the Fall is not the only source of sickness even though that was the gateway in. The effect was far reaching, affecting the animal kingdom also.

CHAPTER 2

The Three Sources of Sickness

As we saw in the last chapter, the effects of the Fall of Man have continued for the last six thousand years, and the reality for everyone is that we all experience sickness to a greater or lesser degree. Even having a vaccination at birth proves the point. We are all vulnerable.

I am going to refer to sickness caused by the Fall and human frailty as physical sickness. For example, that was why Paul left Trophimas sick at Miletus (2 Timothy 4:20) and urged Timothy to take a little wine for his stomach's sake (1 Timothy 5:23). Basically he told him to stop drinking only water because the alcohol killed germs and water in hot countries is suspect. At this juncture I want to make a point which I am convinced is biblically correct and is also the key to knowing how to deal with sickness. There is a clear distinction between sicknesses which are **physical** in nature and origin and those which are **spiritual**. There is a third category where God Himself inflicts disease as a punishment on either individuals or a nation, and we will study those for the sake of completeness. If, like Herod, you take glory for yourself and are struck with worms (Acts 12:23) you won't get better by seeing the doctor. The cure will be good old-fashioned repentance before God!

The three sources of sickness can be simply stated as:

1. The Fall – physical
2. Satan – spiritual
3. God – judgement

We will now see how Satan, the devil, the father of lies, the accuser of the brethren, Apollyon, the destroyer, the dragon etc., fits into the picture.

As in Milton's *Paradise Lost* it's back to Genesis where it all started to go wrong. The physical decay was, of course, God's judgement on Adam and the whole human race, but Adam had more than a body. He had a spirit, which died the moment he sinned, and a soul. He therefore experienced three areas of change: sickness in his body; death in his human spirit; and bondage in his soul. But worst by far was that he was cut off from his fellowship with God. He was exposed, vulnerable and frightened. Suddenly he was now in the middle of a spiritual battle for the future of mankind itself. Satan (Lucifer) had been thrown down onto the earth (Isaiah 14:12) from his position in the heavens, with a third of the angels, and was out to destroy God's creation. The story can be read in Genesis 3, so I only want to draw attention to the consequences of the Fall where they affected Adam and Eve's souls.

First of all their eyes were opened. What does this mean? Clearly they could see physically, but suddenly they could see spiritually also. They were aware of the whole spiritual dimension, which hitherto God had kept from them. They had, as it were, been blind to it. Now they realised they were naked. Innocence was gone forever. Some areas of the spirit realm are out of bounds for everyone. These are most commonly called 'occult' (or hidden) and anyone who strays into these areas, intentionally or not, will be affected, possibly with physical sickness, as we shall see.

From awareness came guilt; from guilt came a covering over to conceal their nakedness; then the passing on of blame.

The attack against Man was on – against his soul, his mind, his will and his emotions. Invisible spirits (demons) would incite, exploit, and, if they could, invade Man's soul. They were using their legal position to execute the curse God had pronounced on Man. Worse, it was possible for these curses to cross generation after generation down through the bloodline.

> *'He by no means clears the guilty, visiting the iniquity of the fathers on the children **to the third and fourth generation.**'*
>
> (Numbers 14:18 NKJV)

It is really important to understand this. We all have two parents, four grandparents, eight great-grandparents, and sixteen great-great-grandparents, making thirty people who affect us spiritually.

The likelihood that they were all godly and righteous saints is somewhat improbable, so there could be a curse which passes on down the family line. Examples would include a high incidence of cancer occurring in the family. Cancer may run in families which, for instance, practise Freemasonry, thus illustrating how it can be passed on spiritually. The incidences of a link between cancer and Freemasonry are far too frequent to ignore or put down as a statistical quirk. That's why Jesus healed the sick (physical) and cast out demons (spiritual), even if they manifested physically as with the woman with the bent back (Luke 13:11).

The text is very clear: she had had a spirit of infirmity for eighteen years, was bent over, and could in no way raise herself up. Jesus told her "*Woman, you are loosed from your infirmity.*" Note that He didn't say healed. It was a spiritual bondage manifesting physically, from which she was released. Jesus made it clear to the ruler of the synagogue when He argued that Satan had bound her. We're not told why, but there was a moment in time eighteen years previously when access was gained by Satan to afflict her body.

I believe it is essential, with God's help, to recognise and discern the root cause of sickness correctly. There are countless cases of people being sick with no apparent medical cause. Doctors often refer to psychosomatic illnesses. That literally means 'disease of the soul' (psyche). It is recognised that well over half of all medical consultations fall into this category! They affect both **soul** and **body**.

The third source of sickness is when God Himself pronounces judgement. This is for those who reject His ways and is the outworking of His curse on mankind. This may sound odd. Indeed people ask how a God of love can do such things. The Deuteronomy 28 covenant with Israel sets out the choices: Obedience and blessing... or... disobedience and cursing. Some of the curses the Jews (God's special chosen people) could receive were plagues (verse 21), consumption/tuberculosis, inflammation and swelling, burning fever (malaria?) (verse 22), boils, tumours (cancer), with the scab and with the itch, from which you cannot be healed (verse 27), madness, blindness, confusion of heart (panic attacks) (verse 29). No use blaming the devil here, or indeed seeing the doctor! It required repentance from their wicked ways. That's still true. God hasn't changed, even if grace is extended because His compassion is over all that He has made (Psalm 145:8-9). Take AIDS, for example. God has immense compassion on men who are so wounded that they desperately seek male friendship and relationship. Yet those who practise an active homosexual lifestyle may receive in their bodies the due **penalty**. Romans 1:27 is clear:

> '... likewise the men... burned with lust for one another; men with men committing what is shameful, and receiving in themselves the **penalty** of their error'

I've heard testimonies of God healing AIDS patients. and I believe it can happen. He is the Almighty and we can draw down His mercy. but if people kept God's laws of monogamous marriage, this problem would disappear. That doesn't mean Christians don't care. Many selflessly devote their lives to teaching, care, and hospice work. The point I'm trying to make is that the answer is good old-fashioned biblical repentance for violating God's laws, not more medical research to protect people from the consequences Romans 1 describes. We break God's laws at our peril.

There are many examples in the Bible of God sending sickness as judgement. The plagues of Egypt would be a clear example. Interestingly barrenness is also attributed to God. '*The Lord closed the womb*' we are told. See Genesis 20:18 (Sarah) and 1 Samuel 5 (Hannah).

We need to understand that God has laws of cause and effect, which operate not just in the natural realm but in the spiritual realm also. We know of many women pronounced medically incapable of conceiving and carrying to full term by the best specialists, yet who are now mothers. How? By identifying the root cause as a curse operating and breaking its power. Indeed I am the godparent of one such child, born after prayer to break the curse of barrenness. The point is simply this. The sickness/problem may be medical (physical). On the other hand it may not be, and if it does have a spiritual root, then by addressing the problem in prayer you may see a dramatic change. I would advise a full medical check first, but especially in cases where there is no apparent cause I would investigate further the possibility of a spiritual cause.

You can be spiritually 100% right with God and still be sick. Elisha had taken on Elijah's mantle, and received the double portion of the Spirit—something we'd all like. He saw Elijah taken up into heaven, yet 2 Kings 13:14 tells us:

'Now Elisha was suffering from the illness from which he died.'

Even the prophet who God had used to heal others was himself equally vulnerable, and subject to the Fall. We need real discernment between the spiritual and the physical, and to check both sources.

CHAPTER 3

The Effects of the Curse

Unfortunately people identify a curse with swearing, when in reality it's the outworking of breaking God's laws, and facing the consequences. The curse works at three levels:

a. On a nation

God's promise to Abraham remains valid (Genesis 12:3). He will curse those who curse Israel, and some nations are in the state they are in because of the way they have treated the Jews over the centuries. That's a whole area you can trace all through history, including Britain's since 1916.

b. On a family

As we've seen earlier, it can run down four generations. That's actually shorter than the curse of illegitimacy which runs for ten generations. In Deuteronomy 23:2 we're told someone with illegitimacy in his line was barred from entering the congregation. Nor were his children allowed in **for ten generations**. Why? Was it fair that children ten generations on paid the price for the sin of others? God says yes, because of the way that curse operates. It is generational in nature. If illegitimacy runs in a family there is a curse operating there, however much sociologists try to validate unbiblical common-law relationships. If there are any sicknesses which 'run in the family' it's living proof of the curse operating. You can read in the newspapers about curses in famous families.

c. On an individual

You may be affected by both the above if you live in a nation opposed to Israel, and come from a family where a hereditary (family) spirit has been wreaking havoc in everyone's lives. In Deuteronomy 27:14-28 the people were told what things would bring a curse into their lives, and they had to say 'Amen' afterwards to show they understood and took it seriously. Galatians 3:10 reinforces this:

'For it is written: "Cursed is everyone who does not continue to do everything written in the Book of the Law".'

The good news for the Christian is that Jesus has freed us from the curse of the Law and we live under grace. For the unbeliever it is not so. They remain under the curse.

However freedom has to be appropriated, like all of the benefits and blessings of salvation. If we remain in the words of Jesus we shall know the truth and the truth shall make us free from every curse operating in our lives. That's an individual's responsibility.

CHAPTER 4
Christ our Redeemer

I hope we can now see the problem! We need to be freed from the effects of the Fall, the Curse, and its consequences. We understand that Jesus died for our sin, but it is essential to understand that He also became a curse for us. By becoming a curse Jesus paid the price for all the effects of the curse upon us and we need to appropriate that redemption by faith.

> `Christ has redeemed us from the curse of the law, having become a curse for us (for it is written "Cursed is everyone who hangs on a tree").'
> (Galatians 3:13 NKJV)

We exchanged our sin and the effects of the sin (the curse) for His righteousness and the effects of it (forgiveness, restoration, health and wholeness).

- That is the key Christians need to know.
- This is the key to health and healing. We are redeemed (bought) from the curse.

Unfortunately the white Western education system of secular humanism denies the reality of such things even existing, but if you're reading this in Africa or Asia you will know immediately the reality of what I'm talking about and the power of curses. Alas, prosperous Western nations deny the reality of the spiritual realm and seek to rationalise everything in purely scientific terms. Jesus spoke of these things a great deal.

I now want to home in on the specifics of how to deal with sickness. This is addressed to the believer. For the unbeliever it's actually different. Indeed it's often easier for God to heal the unbeliever than the believer! Why? Because God will extend grace and mercy to show the unbeliever that he is loved, and that the gospel is true. In other words it's 'power evangelism'; preaching the gospel with signs following to prove it is true, and bringing sinners to repentance. That's why in Mark 16 the disciples and early believers were told to do just that: *'heal the sick... cast out demons'*. It's why people came to Jesus, and it should be why people come to us as well. That's why we hear of spectacular miracles at mass evangelistic rallies. I have seen it myself in India, with lepers healed, paralytics walking, the deaf hearing and the dumb speaking. And these people were Hindus! That's the power of healing and is, I believe, an important part of evangelism. The world is tired of philosophy and religion. They want to see something real and true, and God will confirm His Word with signs **following** the preaching of the Word. That's why I think every healing service needs to have the gospel preached first, so the signs (healing etc.) can follow! It brings faith and honours God.

However, for the believing Christian God paradoxically requires more. He requires repentance, changed behaviour and forgiveness of others. The rules are not the same as for the unbeliever. So we have unconditional power healing for the unbeliever to lead him to repentance, yet healing for the believer is often conditional.

For example, if I regard iniquity in my heart the Lord will not hear me (Psalm 66:18), and indeed 1 Peter 3:7 makes it clear that if you're in contention with your wife your prayers will be hindered.

Too often believers expect God to just ignore their sin, their attitudes and their behaviour, and heal them even when they violate the most basic principles of repentance, faith, forgiveness of others, etc.

Wrong thinking like this leads to disappointment and discredits the gospel. A basic starting point when we go to meetings should be to be totally right with God and one another. God requires us to walk in the light — no skeletons in the cupboard, and to walk in truth — no deception of others, or indeed ourselves. Openness is required.

> *'Confess your sins to one another and pray for one
> another that you may be healed.'*
>
> (James 5:16)

If every healing meeting had a confession time first, I'm sure we'd see more people healed. We cannot ignore the Scriptures and simply hope God will be nice to us if He's in a good mood, or it's a good day for the preacher. Even if you get healed through faith operating, it'll be very hard to retain it.

How many people suffer from arthritis because they will not forgive?

How many people are sick due to bad relationships? Relationships have to be put right. Indeed, Jesus says they have to be put right **before** going to church, and **before** coming into the presence of God.

> *'Therefore, if you are offering your gift at the altar
> and there remember that your brother has something
> against you, leave your gift there in front of the altar.
> First go and be reconciled to your brother; then come
> and offer your gift.'*
>
> (Matthew 5:23-24)

It is that important. You cannot offer up an acceptable sacrifice of praise while others have things against you that you know about and need to be put right. Only then will you really have the boldness and assurance of faith to ask what you want of God with a clean heart (Hebrews 10:19-22).

In most churches there are usually a number of unresolved relationship difficulties, which could block healing.

God wants to deal with the cause, not just the effect. It's your soul He wants to heal, as well as your body. So we need to see what's physical and what's spiritual, and the root cause.

CHAPTER 5

Physical or Spiritual?

To begin with we need to affirm the totality of our salvation (sozo), that Jesus died for every sin of every person, and His sacrifice fully paid the price. We are truly redeemed from every sin, every sickness, every curse, and we need to understand the glory, the fullness and the totality of what God in Christ did for us. It is truly awesome; not just dealing with the sin problem but far, far more. We are ransomed, healed, restored and forgiven. Amazing grace indeed! If Jesus had not redeemed us from the Curse, or indeed died for our sickness, which is a result of the Fall, our salvation would be incomplete. The name Jesus in Hebrew actually means **God heals** as well as **God saves**. His very name proclaims His victory over sickness. If you believe in Jesus you believe in '**God heals**'. That's His name. It's truly marvellous.

In His role as the second Adam He restored all that was lost, even if we do not yet see all the benefits of that restoration here and now on earth.

Hebrews 2:8 tells us:

*'For in that He put all in subjection under Him (Jesus), He left nothing that is not put under him. But now we do not **yet** see all things put under him. But we see Jesus.'*

(NKJV)

In other words, although everything is under the Lord's feet, it's not all yet fully revealed. We have to wait (Romans 8:22-25).

Some physical sicknesses will be obvious, including accidents, broken bones, birth deformities, colds, flu etc. A very good rule of thumb is this: if it's a medically recognised treatable condition it most likely has a straight physical cause. God has physical laws for the human body for our welfare and protection. The human body is designed to heal itself. It has antibodies; and we are indeed fearfully and wonderfully made (Psalm 139:14).

If you are permanently disabled through an accident, your body may be unable to heal itself. You may need a special creative miracle by God. I recently heard of a recreated knee joint, which totally baffled the specialists as the old X-rays showed irreparable damage but the new one showed a perfect knee.

God's will is that we are well, and He uses His physical laws to achieve that. Most medical sicknesses now are curable with a few exceptions, which include viruses, and the common cold. Sick Christians sometimes give up too quickly, assuming it must be God's will that they're sick. That flows from wrong reasoning, which says that God is sovereign, therefore God's will is always done. I'm sick, so that must be God's will. Wrong! The flaw in the argument is that God's will is always done. That is just not so. God's will is that everyone is saved and that none should perish as 2 Peter 3:9 clearly tells us. But clearly many will. So God's will is not done, in that sense. Yes, He remains sovereign, but works within spiritual laws. That's also true of healing.

Some who assert it's God's will for them to be sick actively seek to get out of God's will – if they really believed it to be so – by seeing their doctor. Of course God wants us to get well. We need to move beyond passive simplistic acceptance of sickness as something we just have to accept and live with.

Spiritual or spirit-based sickness is harder to pinpoint. For example headaches can be either, as can migraine, backache, stomach pain and, what in India they call 'body weakness': they just feel ill all over!

However a number of spirit-based diseases are mentioned in the Bible:

A spirit of infirmity (Luke 13:11)

This is a demonic attack of a non-specific sickness. If something is around you get it. Doctors can't identify any cause. You're sickness-prone and it's one thing after another. Alas it's all too common. The most common manifestations are backache and oppressive headaches. There has to be a gateway in for it to operate.

A spirit of heaviness (Isaiah 61:3)

Also called depression. It can be medically caused, as in post-natal depression, and it's estimated that 20% of the population may have a chemical imbalance affecting behaviour, but here we're talking about a spirit bringing that heavy weight of oppression, darkness, suicidal thoughts etc. Jesus quotes this passage in Luke 4. If you discern the cause is demonic, encourage the sufferer to fill their house with the sounds of praise. Their spirit will be fed and the oppression should lift, just as it did when David played for King Saul.

Familiar spirits (Leviticus 19:31)

These run through families and have knowledge of past family members. They operate with psychic powers. Some people mistakenly believe these powers are from God. Others go to spiritualist 'churches' where familiar spirits operate.

Other spirits mentioned are an unclean spirit (Mark 1:23), a dumb spirit (Mark 9:17), a spirit of divination (Acts 16:16), as well as more general references to evil spirits.

So how do you tell? You need the gift of discernment, and to ask God for a word of knowledge or a word of wisdom as to why someone is ill. An evangelist told me about a lady who was constantly sick. He prayed and asked God why the lady remained sick and was told 'It's the water'. The lady got a water filter and couldn't believe what it filtered out. It was like frogspawn. After that she recovered quite quickly. It was a straight problem of poisons and toxins in her water, revealed by a word of knowledge. God really does know the answer.

In her case they started thinking it was a spiritual attack, but God showed it was physical, and the opposite can also be true. We mustn't jump to conclusions. We need wisdom from above to discern correctly, based on the presenting problem.

Chapter 6

Biblical Methods of Healing

Although Jesus used many different methods of healing, from just speaking the word to making paste for a man's eyes, I believe there are three main methods given to the Church.

a. The Laying on of hands

This is based on Mark 16, and is, I believe, for unbelievers as well, repeating the ministry of Jesus.

The promise is that they shall recover. This is important as it implies a process of time. An instant healing is more accurately the working of a miracle. It's important to differentiate to avoid an unbiblical expectation.

The first time I received prayer for a longstanding condition I felt nothing specific change. Nor was I better the next day. But over a 6 week period the condition cleared up and hasn't recurred for 40 years. That's biblical healing — over time. Sometimes I meet someone who asks me if I remember praying for them 6 months ago. They then tell me they are healed now. These were not conditions which would have got better, they were major longstanding illnesses! Wait for God to complete the work, and for full recovery.

b. Summoning the Elders

I believe the pattern in the Church should be:

1. Consult your doctor. There is nothing unspiritual in this. Take whatever medicine is prescribed.

2. At the same time pray for yourself. Ask God to show you why you are sick and how He intends to heal you.

3. If you're still not better after i) and ii) get others to pray for you, such as those in your house group.

If you're still not getting better apply James 5:14 and get your elders to anoint you with oil.

They are not an emergency service to rush round immediately, but are there to pray for you as God's order and remedy.

Note again, it's the prayer of faith, linked to forgiveness of sins. You should have confessed all sins to God and thoroughly repented before you send for the elders. Verse 16 is as important as verse 15.

c. Gifts of healing/special meetings

God has given gifts into the Body of Christ, but believers must go to those meetings properly prepared to receive. These meetings are the preferred route of many, judging by attendance. We want God's man of faith and power and anointing to do it all. It's what I call the Naaman expectation. He was angry when told to do something. It wasn't what he'd come for.

> *'Indeed I said to myself, "He will surely come out to me, and stand and call on the name of the Lord his God, and wave his hand over the place, and heal the leprosy".'*
>
> (2 Kings 5:11)

Is that your expectation? Has God told you to do something? I know of a businessman who wouldn't pay a debt he owed. When he got into the healing line God gave the evangelist a word of knowledge. His refusal to pay was blocking his healing. He went away, paid the debt and was healed. There's a lesson there.

I'm personally keen on special meetings, but they must be done biblically. There must be teaching on repentance, confession, forgiving one another and being in right relationships. That paves way for gifts of healing to flow unhindered, with words of knowledge, plus faith.

We must go properly prepared to really benefit from such meetings, being right with God and right with each other.

A good question to ask is: Is there any reason why God would not want to heal me? Is there anything I need to confess or put right first?

Chapter 7

Blockages to Healing

It's clear we're part of the fallen human race, and we're decaying day by day. But God has redeemed us and given us the firstfruits of a glorious inheritance.

It's not a question of just claiming the promises or rebuking the devourer, but rather discerning what's happening and pulling down those strongholds and every power that would oppose God.

There can be real strongholds to overcome. The most common are:

Unforgiveness and resentment

Many sick people have been really hurt emotionally. They are wounded and all churned up inside. This will manifest in all sorts of ways from stress to rashes to blood conditions to arthritis. I believe such people need God's help to forgive. Yes, the Bible tells us we must forgive others to receive God's forgiveness, and unforgiveness is a blockage. It may take time. If you identify with this I would suggest first focusing prayer on the hurt, then on the sickness. Don't let it take root (Hebrews 12:15).

Occult strongholds

If you have violated major spiritual laws and entered forbidden satanic territory there can be a terrible price to pay. But once you're saved you have the right to be totally free from the effects of these areas, if you have repented and renounced them. This needs to be done before healing prayer. We must verbally renounce all occultic ties, laying the axe to the root.

That includes horoscopes, Ouija boards, fortune telling, tarot cards and even some artifacts in the home which may be picked up innocently. Anything ungodly must be removed. From experience I would include prayer for demonic tattoos, and New Age and occultic jewellery, however fashionable.

Hereditary Curses

We have covered familiar spirits operating in a family, through the bloodline. Does anything run in your family? Cancer? Freemasonry? Heart attacks? Divorce? Miscarriages? Barrenness? In my case it was Christian Science and heart attacks. We need to repent and renounce all involvement, wilful or not.

Unbelief/wrong teaching

If Jesus could do nothing in Nazareth because of unbelief we're unlikely to do any better, and there's a lot about! Wrong teaching and exaggerated claims have created false expectations. Solid biblical teaching will release faith.

> `Paul, observing him intently and **seeing he had faith to be healed**, said with a loud voice "Stand up straight on your feet."!'
>
> (Acts 14:9 NKJV)

Sometimes in the healing line it's right to ask someone 'Do you have faith?' If the answer is not really, then pray for the gift of faith (1 Corinthians 12:9). I've seen that produce healing more effectively than praying irrespectively. God will not work in unbelief. Whatever is not of faith is sin (Romans 14:23) and God will not work other than in the faith realm.

God does not want to block our healing. So if it's not appearing it's quite reasonable to ask why! Words of knowledge and gifts of discernment are there for the Church to be able to overcome these obstacles and see the results we all want.

CHAPTER 8

What to do if You're Sick

- Identify what sickness you have and its likely cause. That may mean consulting your doctor to get a proper diagnosis.

- Get proper treatment and co-operate by taking any medication you are prescribed.

- At the same time pray and ask God to show you if your sickness is caused by any other factor than the basic fall of mankind, and a recognition that we are all in bondage to decay and the ageing process.

For example, are you discerning the body and blood of the Lord Jesus Christ correctly? (1 Corinthians 11:29). Paul tells the believers that because they are doing it in an unworthy manner, i.e. without having repented properly, they are bringing judgement on themselves in the form of sickness. As **many** were sick and some had died, it was clearly a common problem. If it was common then, we cannot discount it now. This is a key passage.

Not discerning the body simply means that you are abusing the fact that Jesus died for you by continuing in wilful sin, and if you continue the result may well be sickness, even sickness unto death (1 Corinthians 11:30).

Persistent refusal to acknowledge sin of any kind and turn away from it may well lead to sickness in varying forms. You must judge sin in your life (1 Corinthians 11:31) or God will do it (verse 30).

It does not necessarily follow that if you're sick that's the reason, but a Christian out of fellowship forfeits God's protection, and I have seen this. I have also seen it in cases where people refuse to heed a prophetic warning from God.

I believe the key is a right relationship with God and with one another. Because we all fall short of God's standard we need to identify areas of spiritual vulnerability and confess and renounce any possible occultic activity and other gateways into our lives including such common practises as fortune-telling and reading horoscopes in the daily newspaper.

However, we're all vulnerable, so what if you're diagnosed with a major illness, potentially terminal? In addition to the above I would suggest a time of prayer and fasting.

There are three things which always touch God's heart: repentance, humility, and fasting. He has a heart of compassion, grace, love and mercy. I firmly believe in the promises of God, but don't like the approach of commanding healing, although I do believe in aggressive praying if it is a demonic attack.

I prefer to ask God for His mercy, grace and healing, not as a 'right', but as a blessing of sonship.

Repentance

This is so fundamental to healing, yet is not included in many meetings. 1 John 1:9 is the key:

'If we confess our sins, He is faithful and just to forgive us our sins and to cleanse us from all unrighteousness.'

(NKJV)

It has two parts – forgiveness **and** cleansing.

God is absolutely faithful to forgive us when we confess our sin. He knows us through and through, but still requires this of us. It will affect how He views us.

Humility

God always notes those who humble themselves. For example, when Ahab was told of judgement he humbled himself.

God actually said to Elijah,

> *'Do you see how Ahab has humbled himself before me? Because he has humbled himself before me I will not bring the calamity in his days'*
>
> (1 Kings 21:29)

God resists the proud but gives grace to the humble.

> *`Therefore humble yourselves under the mighty hand of God'*
>
> (1 Peter 5:5-6)

Humility gets God's attention.

Fasting

In Isaiah 58:6-8 God describes the fast He's looking for. Please read it if you're sick! The conclusion is:

> *`Then shall your light break forth like the morning,* **your healing shall spring forth speedily.***'*
>
> (Isaiah 59:8)

There is a fast for healing. We can influence God!

Jesus said we should never give up. Keep praying, keep asking, keep knocking.

Jesus is the same yesterday, today, and forever (Hebrews 13:8) and divine healing definitely didn't cease with the early Church. Indeed testimonies run all through Church history.

Should everyone be healed? I believe that is possible if we had all the knowledge, all the keys, and all the faith. Sometimes God's answer is no, as with Paul's thorn in the flesh, but he got his answer from God. We need to know the mind of the Lord, but until God specifically says no (and Paul was given the reason), then I believe we should continue to pray and expect to get better. We should appeal to God for His mercy.

The principles outlined above are well illustrated in 2 Kings chapter 20. Hezekiah was sick. Actually he was going to die.

Isaiah told him,

> *"Thus saith the Lord; 'Set You house in order, for **you shall die**, and not live'."*
> (Verse 1)

That was a definite word from God.
But Hezekiah turned his face to the wall and prayed:

> *"'Remember now, O Lord, I pray, how I have walked before you in your sight.' And Hezekiah wept bitterly."*

That touched God's heart. God changed His mind! Isaiah hadn't left the premises before God told him:

> *"Return and tell Hezekiah... I have heard your prayer, I have seen your tears; surely **I will heal you**."*

God added 15 years to his life. Hezekiah had touched God's heart. Note he went the medical route for his boil with a poultice of figs. No 'instant' healing there, but it is well worth studying the route Hezekiah took to obtain his healing. A good model is:

1. Confess all known sin.

2. Repent and renounce anything which you think might have caused the sickness.

3. Remind God of your service to Him.

4. Appeal to God's mercy, love and grace.

David writes in Psalm 103:

'Bless the Lord, O my soul.
And forget not all his benefits:
Who forgives all your iniquities,
*Who **heals all your diseases**.'*

He knew what we need to know. Right relationship with God and one another opens the way for God to work powerfully in our lives bringing maximum blessing and health.

Finally remember that the name **Jesus** means **God heals**. It's His name and it's His nature. He wants to do it for you.

'Call on Me in the day of trouble:
I will deliver you, and you shall glorify Me.'

(Psalm 50:15)

That's for this life. But for eternity God has promised us a new resurrection body. Paul describes this in 1 Corinthians 15. No more sickness, no more pain. Truly we shall be like Jesus, healed in spirit, soul, and body.

Chapter 9

Finally... never give up

Sometimes it all seems so unfair. We've tried our best to serve God, yet still we're sick. We are basically people of faith, who trust in the Lord, yet may have an ongoing debilitating condition. What should we do? God is good, yet it can seem to us that He is not giving us the answer we need.

In Luke 18, Jesus told His disciples a parable to show them that they should **always pray and never give up**. He said:

> *"In a certain town there was a judge who neither feared God nor cared about men, And there was a widow in that town who kept coming to him with the plea, 'Grant me justice against my adversary.'*
>
> *"For some time he refused. But finally he said to himself, 'Even though I don't fear God or care about men, yet because this widow keeps bothering me I will see that she gets justice, so that she won't eventually wear me out with her coming.'*
>
> *"And the Lord said, 'Listen to what the unjust judge says. And will not God bring about justice for his chosen ones, who cry out to him day and night? Will he keep putting them off? I tell you, he will see that they get justice and quickly'."*

We need to invest our faith in praying positively and persistently to our Father in heaven, and never give up.

2 Peter 3:7 reminds us:

"The Lord is not slow in keeping his promise, as some understand slowness."

It may take time, but we need to keep praying, particularly in the context of a church, where believers can bear one another's burdens. Jesus presences Himself in the midst, and we can apply the Word of God:

"Is any one of you in trouble? He should pray. Is anyone happy? Let him sing songs of praise. Is any one of you sick? He should call the elders of the church to pray over him and anoint him with oil in the name of the Lord. ***And the prayer offered in faith will make the sick person well; the Lord will raise him up.*** *If he has sinned he will be forgiven.*
Therefore confess your sins to each other and ***pray for each other so that you may be healed.****"*
(James 5:14)

May the Word of God and faith bring you the healing you need. in the name of Jesus, whose very name means '***God heals***'. Amen

CHAPTER 10

For Me to Live is Christ, to Die is Gain

(Philippians 1:21)

Can you say that? Is death something that is better for you than this life?

Paul was able to, because he knew who he had believed and was persuaded that nothing could separate him from the love of God. His knowledge and revelation of Jesus was such that he not only didn't fear death but welcomed it. He lived for Christ, but to be with Him was gain, i.e. far better.

Now we all want to see our children grow up, and indeed their children too. I am not recommending an early death for anyone, but what I am saying is that it is totally different for Christians than unbelievers, who the Bible describes as 'having no hope' (1 Thessalonians 4:13).

If you have any fear of death read 1 Corinthians 15:54-55 where Paul describes how the sting of death is gone for the believer and death is swallowed up in victory. It's not going to sting you if you have trusted in Christ as your saviour.

Personally, my favourite verse on this is Job 19:25:

I know that my Redeemer lives,
And He shall stand at last on the earth:
And after my skin is destroyed, this I know,
That in my flesh I shall see God,
Whom I shall see for myself, and my eyes shall
*   behold, and not another.*
How my heart yearns within me!   (NKJV)

Does your heart yearn within you? The Holy Spirit stirs me every time I read this, and I shall ask for Handel's Messiah, not all of it(!), but the part...

I KNOW THAT MY REDEEMER LIVETH

... to be played at my funeral! I want those there to know that I know this through and through and God will give me the greatest gift He could give anyone, salvation through Jesus Christ. I do believe in divine healing – passionately, but I also believe that there is a time for every purpose under heaven, a time to be born and a time to die (Ecclesiastes 3:2). The key is not to die before your time and to fulfil all that God has called you to do, but when that time does come, Jesus will be there for you.

If you have received a diagnosis of a life threatening illness pray and never give up (Luke 18:3-8), but it honestly isn't the end of your world. At the very worst it's an early entry into the next one, and it's those left behind who grieve, not you. Of course that's hard for them, especially children, but we do need the revelation of the bigger picture of God's eternal plan for us, including a new heaven and new earth for redeemed man.

Death is not the end for the Christian, and the Bible describes it as falling asleep (Acts 7:60, 1 Corinthians 15:6 and 18).

However many times God heals you, and for me it's been a lot, nevertheless our ultimate destination is to be with Him forever. God wants us with Him.

> *"Precious in the sight of the LORD is the death of His saints."*
>
> (Psalm 116:15)

Meanwhile may you know the abundant life Jesus came to bring, full salvation AND full health (sozo), in the name of Jesus which means 'God heals'.

The two big challenges are sickness/healing and God's financial provision. We will now address the question of prosperity.

CHAPTER 11

What is Prosperity?

"A man's life does not consist in the abundance of things he possesses."
Jesus
(Luke 12:15)

Introduction

This teaching, previously called *Explaining Prosperity*, is reproduced here to help you understand that God will provide for all your needs but does not promise to go beyond that!

Prosperity—what could be better for any person? Money, health, the good life, a nice home, car, foreign holidays—it all sounds too good to be true. Is this really what God wants for all His children? Or have we interpreted God's promises to mean what we expect and want, and what our natural senses desire? In all the many meetings I've attended over 40 years I have yet to hear a call to come forward to be poor and sick! So what does God promise us, and what should every believer be in faith for?

I believe that the Word of God applies to all people, in all cultures, at all times in history, in all circumstances, from the farmer in India to the factory worker in China, and that all Christians should be experiencing the abundant life that Jesus came to bring. Wherever you are while reading this, it applies to you!

"I have come that they may have life, and that they may have it more abundantly."
(John 10:10)

More means more. God wants us to have a much better, fuller, richer and more abundant life than we would ever have without Christ. It's as if Jesus says He came to give life, not just eternal life, but life here on earth in abundance. Is that possible? Is it right? What should we expect in a world clearly divided between rich and poor at every level, international, national, local and even in the church?

Biblical principles

The best way of studying any subject is with an oversight of biblical principles, plus a detailed look at words which define the subject, from a concordance. I would like to attempt a definition of prosperity as 'living in the grace, mercy and abundant provision of God to meet all my needs, and to have an abundant overflow to meet the needs of others'.

In other words it covers all my needs, not just financial ones, but in every area of my life. After all, the richest man in the world, John Paul Getty, is reputed to have replied to the question as to whether all his money had made him happy, "money helps you to be miserable in comfort". That's hardly abundant life. Indeed, abundant life cannot even begin without being born again and being in right relationship with God. That is a key, and when the Bible uses terms like 'wealth' or 'prosperity', or 'it will go well with you', it's always in the context of a right walk with God, and obedience to His commands.

On the positive side you have verses like 1 Chronicles 22:11-13, given to Solomon:

> *"Now, my son, may the Lord be with you; and may you prosper; build the house of the Lord your God, as He has said to you. Only may the Lord give you wisdom and understanding, and give you charge concerning Israel, that you may keep the law of the Lord your God. Then you will prosper, if you take care to fulfill the statutes and judgments with which the Lord charged Moses concerning Israel."*
>
> (NKJV)

Note that it's **if** you take care to fulfil God's commands. On the negative side you have Proverbs 28:13:

"He who covers his sins will not prosper"

Yet God continues to give the solution:

"But whoever confesses and forsakes them will have mercy."

So the precondition of prosperity has to be living with our sins confessed to God, living in repentance, i.e. turning around and going in the opposite direction, and experiencing God's grace and mercy.

So the first and greatest need we have is forgiveness of sins and right standing with God. Although we are partakers of a new covenant of grace and mercy (Hebrews 8:6), nevertheless the old covenant tells us about the character and nature of an unchanging God. In Deuteronomy 29:9 Moses tells the people:

"Therefore keep the words of this covenant, and do them, that you may prosper in all you do."

(verse 1)

The covenant he refers to is spelt out in Deuteronomy 28, and is, I believe, the key to prosperity in every area of our lives, even though we live under a new and 'better' covenant of mercy, grace and forgiveness. Nevertheless the same principle, that obedience leads to blessing, is firmly stated here.

"If you diligently obey the voice of the Lord your God... all these blessings shall come upon you..."

Note it is conditional. *If* you **diligently** obey.

Because we live in a world of self-choice we can lack the discipline to be diligent, or worse, do what we like, and claim that because we're no longer under the law but grace, it's O.K. It isn't, because the fact that God forgives you does not of itself excuse any sin, if the Bible clearly places a requirement on a believer. For example, when Paul writes "let the thief no longer steal", you can't just continue to steal and say, "I'm living in God's grace"! If we want the blessings we have to fulfil the core condition of obedience to the Word of God.

The Blessings of God

The main blessings are listed in Deuteronomy 28:2-13:

"And all these blessings shall come upon you and overtake you, because you obey the voice of the Lord your God."

(verse 2)

You get them because you obey the voice of the Lord your God. The blessings listed are all-encompassing:

"Blessed shall you be in the city and blessed shall you be in the country."

(verse 3)

"Blessed shall be the fruit of your body, the produce of your ground and the increase of your herds, the increase of your cattle and the offspring of your flocks."

(verse 4)

"Blessed shall be your basket and your kneading bowl."

(verse 5)

"Blessed shall you be when you come in, and blessed shall you be when you go out."

(verse 6)

"The Lord will cause your enemies who rise against you to be defeated before your face; they shall come out against you one way and flee before you seven ways."

(verse 7)

"The Lord will command the blessing on you in your store-houses and in all to which you set your hand, and He will bless you in the land which the Lord your God is giving you."

(verse 8)

"The Lord will establish you as a holy people to Himself just as He has sworn to you, if you keep the commandments of the Lord your God and walk in His ways."

(verse 9)

"Then all peoples of the earth shall see that you are called by the name of the Lord, and they shall be afraid of you."

(verse 10)

"And the Lord will grant you plenty of goods, in the fruit of your body, in the increase of your livestock, and in the produce of your ground, in the land of which the Lord swore to your fathers to give you."

(verse 11)

"The Lord will open to you His good treasure, the heavens, to give the rain to your land in its season, and to bless all the work of your hand. You shall lend to many nations, but you shall not borrow."

(verse 12)

"And the Lord will make you the head and not the tail; you shall be above only and not be beneath, if you heed the commandments of the Lord your God, which I command you today, and are careful to observe them."

(verse 13)

If you heed the commandments, you will be in charge, in control and on top of every area of your life. What a promise!

Then from verse 15 onwards the curses are listed. The blessings are covered in fourteen verses, while the curses take fifty-three verses – over four times as long. God was really spelling out the choices and the consequences in great detail. We disobey the Word of God at our peril. The covenant expresses God's heart. The blessings fall into three main categories.

Work

Expect God's favour and blessing in your work area, whether you work with your brain (city) or with your hands (country). In other words, every area of business – commerce, industry, farming, teaching, etc.

Family and relationships

Expect blessing in your family as you establish God's order. Other principles in the Word of God need to be applied, as the promise doesn't work independently of other biblical principles.

Control of your affairs

The prosperity will give you financial stability through the increase which God sends through whichever area of endeavour you are involved in.

Because Man has fallen, it's just like our salvation, i.e. some is for now, some for the future, and not everyone's circumstances allow all of the blessings to flow in their lives immediately. Nevertheless this was what God had in mind for His obedient people, and it expresses His heart towards us, one of blessing and abundance. We need to press into it.

The real point about the Deuteronomy 28 covenant is that it shows that prosperity and blessing go beyond money and health to a total well-being, peace and security. At a national level, if the Jewish people had kept the covenant, God would indeed have made them the head and not the tail, and the leading nation on earth, instead of a dispossessed, despised people unsafe in other countries, as history records.

Prosperity in the New Testament

If we are truly redeemed from the curse of the Law (Galatians 3:13) then how does this affect a believer today? Are the blessings our birthright? My Young's Concordance gives only two references to prosperity in the New Testament, but 88 in the Old Testament, where the link between obedience and prosperity/wellbeing is so clearly defined.

The two New Testament references are:

1. A reference to Christian giving.

> *"On the first day of the week let each one of you lay something aside, storing up as he may prosper."*
> (1 Corinthians 16:2 NKJV)

Clearly it is proportionate. Not everyone will have an equal income, so according to how you prosper, Paul instructs setting aside an indeterminate amount to fund the ministry on a weekly basis. Rather than having separate collections, planned giving is encouraged, based on your income. If you're paid weekly give every week; if you're paid monthly, do it monthly.

2. A greeting from John's third letter.

> *"Beloved, I pray that you may prosper in all things and be in health, just as your soul prospers."*
> (3 John 2 NKJV)

It was a normal greeting of the time, rather like saying 'Your good health' as a toast, and should not be taken as a major theological basis for teaching that John wanted them to *'prosper and be in health'* as a top priority, as he goes on to say he has no greater joy than to hear that *'my children walk in truth'*, i.e. obedience to the Word of God. Those who would make a 'health and wealth' doctrine out of this risk being sorely disappointed as it just doesn't carry that emphasis in the New Testament. It's rather like the claim I heard an evangelist make at a meeting, where he seriously claimed that the reason Peter and John said *"silver and gold have I none"* was because they were not in the revelation of divine prosperity! There is no other/higher revelation than the Word of God available to us which supersedes the New Testament. The New Testament emphasis is a sacrificial life, taking up your cross and following Jesus. Having said that it's a nice greeting of blessing. Today we might say 'I trust the Lord is blessing you, and you're in good health'. How nice to be met with a greeting like that.

Prosperity or well-being in the New Testament is not primarily a social or economic measure, rather it is a spiritual measure of the blessings of God. Money scarcely comes into it. I love the way Solomon in the Proverbs defines where to aim:

> *"Give me neither poverty nor riches – lest I be full and deny You, and say 'Who is the Lord?' or lest I be poor and steal, and profane the name of my God."*
>
> (Proverbs 30:8-10 NKJV)

What good advice from a multi-millionaire of his day! How many Christians are praying that God won't give them too much, lest they forget Him and no longer need to live by faith? It's more likely they are praying for a pay increase! Paul also writes:

> *"I have learned in whatever state I am in to be content."*
>
> (Philippians 4:11)

He had to **learn** to be content in the ups and downs of life. The same message is repeated to Timothy:

> *"And having food and clothing with these we shall be content"*
>
> (1 Timothy 6:6-8)

He then warns what a snare the love of money is, even to believers, in very clear terms in verse 10.

> *"For the love of money is the root of all kinds of evil, for which some have strayed from the faith in their greediness, and pierced themselves through with many sorrows."*
>
> (NKJV)

The love of money was and still is a big snare for believers. So if prosperity isn't money, what precisely is it and how do you get it?

I defined it earlier as 'living in the grace, mercy, and abundant provision of God to meet all my needs, and to have an overflow to meet the needs of others.'

This encompasses my relationship with God, with my family, with the church, with other believers, with those I work with, and with those in the world. If I can be blessed in all those areas, life will be good indeed. The good news is that as it is not money-dependent, it's available for all believers, with however little they may have.

Having said that, money does matter, because our attitude to it will affect our attitude to so much else. Indeed, God requires good stewardship of us, and if we are obedient and faithful in whatever we have, God can then add His increase to us and know He can trust us with it.

> *"He who is faithful in what is least is faithful also in much; and he who is unjust in what is least is unjust also in much. "Therefore if you have not been faithful in the unrighteous mammon (money), who will commit to your trust the true riches?"*
>
> (Luke 16:10-11)

Note, God sees how you handle money as the basis of whether you're trustworthy with a ministry, and spiritual gifts!

Wealth—relative and absolute

When you read about the super-rich, those whose personal fortune is hundreds of millions of dollars, that is absolute wealth. It's basically far more than they could need, use or spend in a lifetime. So much of it gets inherited by the next generation, and so on. Relative wealth is defined by the per capita income of a country. We have, wisely or not, divided up countries into three worlds.

1. The First World or 'Western World', even if it includes Australia and New Zealand! These are mainly free-market economies on a capitalist model of economic management, and would include places like Singapore. They overflow with everything from mobile phones to computers to high-tech products like cars and satellite TV's.

2. The Second World, mainly Eastern European and Communist countries, with a much lower per capita income, run mainly on a Socialist command economy model. Many are now trying to get into First World economic management, for example by joining the European Union. It also includes 'emerging economies' in South America and Asia. A small elite may have First World life styles. Most don't. Technology and investment lags behind the West.

3. The Third World, or developing nations, mainly still agricultural economies, some with subsistence living, and underdeveloped political structures, e.g. they could be a dictatorship in all but name, as with many African countries with military rulers. There is often a shortage of goods, and electricity may go on and off at random. My observation in visiting many Second and Third World countries is that the believers there are generally far more radiant, content, grateful and full of love for God than their brothers and sisters in the West. I have seen offerings where an egg or handful of rice was given out of real gratitude to God. The widow's mite indeed.

So economic prosperity as a nation isn't the same as personal prosperity, God meeting your needs, and being content. Paul writes in 1 Timothy 6:6-8:

> *"With food and clothing, with these we shall be content."*

If you took that definition we should never hear another grumble from any believer alive and wearing clothes!

Clearly poverty means different things in different countries. In the U.K. it means not having a television or a refrigerator or even a telephone. These days you can claim a fridge on welfare as a 'basic need'.

In Africa it may mean having very little food, and to have a house with a corrugated iron roof would be considered prosperity indeed. Yet God loves all these people the same and wants to see the believers manifest His glory through their stewardship, and abundant life.

So does the Bible see wealth as a good thing or not? Should believers expect it and aim for it, or simply accept their lot in life? I believe that God wants to bless in this area, because, as a Father, it expresses His provision.

What we have to do is be obedient and fulfil the conditions to embrace the blessing, but it may not come in the form of money alone.

> *"Praise the Lord! Blessed is the man who fears the Lord,*
> *Who delights greatly in His commandments.*
> *His descendants will be mighty on the earth;*
> *The generation of the upright will be blessed.*
> *Wealth and riches will be in his house,*
> *And his righteousness endures forever.*
> *Unto the upright there arises light in the darkness;*
> *He is gracious, and full of compassion, and righteous.*
> *A good man deals graciously and lends;*
> *He will guide his affairs with discretion.*
> *Surely he will never be shaken;*
> *The righteous will be in everlasting remembrance.*

He will not be afraid of evil tidings;
His heart is steadfast, trusting in the Lord.
His heart is established;
He will not be afraid,
Until he sees his desire upon his enemies.
He has dispersed abroad,
He has given to the poor;
His righteousness endures forever;
His horn will be exalted with honor."

(Psalm 112:1-9 NKJV)

"And you shall remember the Lord your God, for it is He who gives you power to get wealth, that He may establish His covenant."

(Deuteronomy 8:18 NKJV)

In other words, if you keep your part, God gives wealth and it establishes His covenant as God the Provider. God wants balance, hard work and His blessing. It is summarised by Solomon:

"Here is what I have seen: It is good and fitting for one to eat and drink, and to enjoy the good of all his labor in which he toils under the sun all the days of his life which God gives him: for it is his heritage.

"As for every man to whom God has given riches and wealth, and given him power to eat of it, to receive his heritage and rejoice in his labor – this is the gift of God."

(Ecclesiastes 5:18-19 NKJV)

Most of us are locked into an economic system over which we have no control. Our income is determined by 'market forces'. Tax is set by the government, interest rates on the mortgage are set by some Central Bank, and promotion may be on the whim of someone higher up the greasy pole! But God knows all this, so He sets out how the believer is to respond. I'd like to suggest some practical ways you can see your income go up and your expenses come down.

As an employee

Be the best you can be. Get any qualifications you can through study at home. Be reliable, be conscientious, be good at your job. Go the extra mile or stay on if asked to without grumbling. Why? Because you represent the gospel and because it is God-honouring.

> "Servants, be obedient to those who are your masters according to the flesh, with fear and trembling, in sincerity of heart, as to Christ; not with eyeservice, as men-pleasers, but as servants of Christ, doing the will of God from the heart, with goodwill doing service, as to the Lord, and not to men, knowing that whatever good anyone does, he will receive the same from the Lord, whether he is a slave or free."
>
> (Ephesians 6:5-8)

In this selfish world you should stand out as honest, reliable, and worthy of promotion. You should get promoted just like Daniel, Hananiah, Mishael and Azariah, through God-given ability and wisdom.

> Then the king interviewed them, and among them all none was found like Daniel, Hananiah, Mishael, and Azariah; therefore they served before the king. And in all matters of wisdom and understanding about which the king examined them, he found them ten times better than all the magicians and astrologers who were in all his realm.
>
> (Daniel 1:19-20 NKJV)

Later on we read how these men, now re-named, refused to compromise on an issue of principle, or yield to King Nebuchadnezzar's anger. God vindicated them and they came out of the fire untouched. They also got promotion. Even unrighteous kings recognise principle and integrity.

> *Nebuchadnezzar spoke, saying, "Blessed be the God of Shadrach, Meshach, and Abed-Nego, who sent His Angel and delivered His servants who trusted in Him, and they have frustrated the king's word, and yielded their bodies, that they should not serve or worship any god except their own God!*
>
> *"Therefore I make a decree that any people, nation, or language which speaks anything amiss against the God of Shadrach, Meshach, and Abed-Nego shall be cut in pieces, and their houses shall be made an ash heap; because there is no other God who can deliver like this."*
>
> *Then the king promoted Shadrach, Meshach, and Abed-Nego in the province of Babylon.*
>
> (Daniel 3:28-30 NKJV)

Daniel himself was promoted further because of his good service to the king, which provoked jealousy, but the king valued him highly.

> *Then this Daniel distinguished himself above the governors and satraps, because an excellent spirit was in him; and the king gave thought to setting him over the whole realm. So the governors and satraps sought to find some charge against Daniel concerning the kingdom; but they could find no charge or fault, because he was faithful; nor was there any error or fault found in him.*
>
> (Daniel 6:3-4 NKJV)

The point is not that you may be thrown into the fiery furnace. The test will most likely be another issue of righteousness within the business. These men represented God and as a result got promoted, because even unbelievers can see goodness and integrity. It challenges them.

Expect promotion, if you want it, and if your business isn't big enough to promote you, then pray about a move. You're sure to get a first class reference if you've served well. Is this wishful thinking? In my own experience going after my first job, God caused me to beat 1,000 other graduates who applied! That has to be God. On another occasion, following a word of prophecy God gave me that I would be as Joseph to Pharaoh, I was promoted to Personal Assistant to the Managing Director.

As an employer

If you want your business to do well you need to apply Colossians 4:1 and ensure you haven't violated James 5:4.

> *"Masters, give your servants what is just and fair, knowing that you also have a Master in heaven."*
>
> (Colossians 4:1)

> *"Indeed the wages of the laborers who mowed your fields, which you kept back by fraud, cry out; and the cries of the reapers have reached the ears of the Lord of Sabbaoth."*
>
> (James 5:4)

A good test is this. Could they earn more elsewhere doing the same job? If so, you may be paying below the proper rate for the job. Even if there are constraints such as how much the firm can afford, or market conditions, nevertheless I do believe that God will bless businesses who act righteously and treat their staff well. They won't want to leave! The true cost of a member of staff is the cost of replacing them. I have personally known and seen this to be true in over 40 years in business.

As a self-employed person

Most self-employed people are small businessmen/craftsmen and it gives them great opportunity for God to bless them. It is, however, the most difficult area to manage. You must be good at your job to get a good reputation, charge a fair price, put right any faults immediately, and do the job when you say you will at the price quoted. My own experience is that this does not always happen, causing believers to wonder why the work has dried up. You live by your reputation, good or bad. Make it a good one.

Also to enjoy the fullness of blessing, you must declare all income, cash or not. Keep proper records, declare an honest income, and pay your tax on time. That may sound like a tall order, but it is God's order, and He doesn't ask us to do anything that we cannot reasonably do.

> *"For because of this you also pay taxes, for they are God's ministers attending continually to this very thing. Render therefore to all their due: taxes to whom taxes are due, customs to whom customs, fear to whom fear, honor to whom honor."*
>
> (Romans 13:6-7 NKJV)

If you want God's blessing/prosperity you have to work His way. The Puritans did this and were held in high esteem by the unbelievers of their day. How can you prosper by fiddling the books, under-declaring your income and being dishonest? It just won't work biblically for you. God cannot bless sin.

In this area look what happened to Jacob in Genesis 30. He was paid in kind, as sheep meant wealth, and God increased Jacob's wealth no matter how many times Laban tried to cheat him. The end result was:

> *"Thus the man became exceedingly prosperous and had large flocks, male and female servants, camels and donkeys."*
>
> (Genesis 30:43 NKJV)

God can cause you to prosper in adverse circumstances, whether as a farmer, a construction worker, a computer consultant or a shopkeeper.

Giving

Prosperity and giving are linked together, because God is a giving God and expects us to give also.

> *"There is one who scatters, yet increases more;*
> *And there is one who withholds more than is right,*
> *but it leads to poverty."*
>
> (Proverbs 11:24-25 NKJV)

Much has been said in recent years about giving and tithing and that we are no longer under Law (compulsion) but under grace (free-will), yet we find in Malachi 3:8 that God complains that the people robbed Him of tithes (compulsory) and offerings (free-will). I used to think that this was extraordinary. If an offering was free-will and therefore non-compulsory, how could you be robbing God? After all, it wasn't a requirement of the Law.

I believe the answer is that we rob God of the chance to bless us as He wants to by either being legalistic and giving strictly 10% and absolutely no more, or by being plain mean. It denies God the chance He wants to **prove** His faithfulness and provision. The best way to cut yourself off from God's provision is to refuse to give to God's work. Many believers do that, and wonder why they can't make ends meet, believing they cannot afford to give.

> *"Yet from the days of your fathers*
> *You have gone away from My ordinances*
> *And have not kept them.*
> *Return to Me, and I will return to You,"*
> *Says the Lord of hosts.*
> *"But you said,*
> *`In what way shall we return?'"*
> *"Will a man rob God?*
> *Yet you have robbed Me!*
> *But you say, 'In what way have we robbed You?'*
> *In tithes and offerings.*
> *You are cursed with a curse,*

For you have robbed Me,
Even this whole nation.
Bring all the tithes into the storehouse,
That there may be food in My house,
And try Me now in this,"
Says the Lord of hosts,
"If I will not open for you the windows of heaven
And pour out for you such blessing
That there will not be room enough to receive it.
And I will rebuke the devourer for your sakes,
So that he will not destroy the fruit of your ground,
Nor shall the vine fail to bear fruit for you in the field,"
Says the Lord of hosts;
"And all nations will call you blessed,
For you will be a delightful land,"
Says the Lord of hosts.

(Malachi 3:7-12 NKJV)

You may wonder what this has to do with prosperity. If we want God's blessing we must keep His requirements, even if we live under grace.

Grace may say that the tithe is no longer compulsory, but even if you believe that all giving is now 'offerings', you can still rob God. That's the point. He requires us to give the firstfruits of our labour and not to look for escape clauses to duck our biblical obligation to give. If you want prosperity you have to be a giver. There are no opt-out clauses.

Expenditure

Governments work out the average 'expenditure' by adding together all the expenditure in the country and dividing it by the population. That gives an 'average' income. It includes everything: alcohol, cigarettes, gambling etc. So if you aren't spending money in these areas you should statistically be better off as a notional amount is included in your income for these activities! If cigarettes go up in price, the cost of living goes up and your income probably goes up, making you better off if you're a non-smoker.

How do you spend your money?

It is perfectly possible to be corrupted on 90% of your income after you tithe, assuming it's now your part to spend as you choose.

Sometimes Christians do get into debt, borrow unwisely, and may need help managing money. I once sent some money to help build a church in India, and the pastor, perhaps unwisely, wrote to thank me for the money which he had spent on his daughter's school fees! I have seen cases where the church has paid off someone's debt, and almost immediately they have gone and borrowed an even larger sum of money. Get proper debt counselling if you are already in debt. If you live beyond your income it creates huge stress and the situation cannot carry on. Get help if you need it.

> *Now godliness with contentment is great gain. For we brought nothing into this world, and it is certain we can carry nothing out. And having food and clothing, with these we shall be content.*
>
> *But those who desire to be rich fall into temptation and a snare,*
>
> *And into many foolish and harmful lusts which drown men in destruction and perdition.*
>
> *For the love of money is a root of all kinds of evil, for which some have strayed from the faith in their greediness, and pierced themselves through with many sorrows.*
>
> (1 Timothy 6:6-10 NKJV)

It was a problem then. It is an even bigger problem now, as we see all the things we'd really like advertised in the media, and our children expect to have what they see others having.

Manipulation in Giving

Beware of being a manipulator or being manipulated yourself. Giving should be free-will, in secret, and in faith, not to try and force God to give it back to you straight away however many-fold. That is why God loves a cheerful giver

(2 Corinthians 9:7), who gives with no strings attached. You will not succeed in manipulating God to give you money.

Equally don't be manipulated by preachers trying to prise money out of you by implying that if you don't give more, you don't love God enough. I have been in meetings where people have pledged up to three years' salary or brought forward to the stage their car keys.

I have seen others told to get out their cheque books and wave them in the air as a wave offering, then write the biggest cheque they have ever written to the speaker's ministry!

If God has told you to do that I'm sure He can wait 24 hours for you to check it by the cold light of day. If you have an ordered life with proper planned giving and good stewardship, then God will bless you. I'm always cautious when the money goes directly to the person who is asking for it. It's different with a church offering to support a pastor, but it is always a danger where money and ministry touch, and there must be proper accountability within the Body of Christ.

Offerings should also be going into the worldwide work of God, not to a few very capable fundraisers on TV. In the U.S.A. 98% of all giving remains in the United States, and the 2% which goes overseas funds 90% of all world missionary work. What a blessing it would be if we even got to a 80/20 split. Then world mission would have ten times what it has now. Money is not to be spent on ourselves but is to be used to support the work of God and your family.

Prosperity for all

Wherever you are reading this book, whether you bought it or were given it, the good news is that God wants you to prosper. You won't get prosperous any other way than by obedience to the Word of God, and fulfilment of God's conditions. We pray routinely in our office that God will show us anything that could block the abundance of His blessing towards us, and we continue to be blessed, sometimes in very difficult conditions. People say "It's alright for you, you're doing well," but a better question would be "Why are you doing so well?" Fundamentally it is because we have made the choice to follow the route of blessing, with all it means, as set out in Deuteronomy 11:26-27:

> *"Behold, I set before you today a blessing and a curse: the blessing, if you obey the commandments of the Lord your God which I command you today; and the curse, if you do not obey the commandments of the Lord your God, but turn aside from the way which I command you today, to go after other gods which you have not known."*
>
> (NKJV)

We see this principle affirmed in Joshua 1 when the Israelites entered the Promised Land.

> *"Only be strong and very courageous, that you may observe to do according to all the law which Moses My servant commanded you; do not turn from it to the right hand or to the left, that you may prosper wherever you go.*
>
> *"This Book of the Law shall not depart from your mouth, but you shall meditate in it day and night, that you may observe to do according to all this is written in it. For then you will make your way prosperous, and then You will have good success."*
>
> (Joshua 1:7-8 NKJV)

David re-affirms it in Psalm 1:

> *Blessed is the man who walks not in the counsel of the ungodly,*
> *Nor stands in the path of sinners,*
> *Nor sits in the seat of the scornful;*
> *But his delight is in the law of the Lord,*
> *And in His law he meditates day and night.*
> *He shall be like a tree planted by the rivers of water,*
> *That brings forth its fruit in its season,*
> *Whose leaf also shall not wither;*

And whatever he does shall prosper.

(Psalm 1:1-3 NKJV)

These men had seen and proved the Word of God. There are no short-cuts, no by-passing God's Word. We need to heed the warning of Zechariah:

> *"Thus says God: 'Why do you transgress the commandments of God, so that you cannot prosper?'"*
>
> (2 Chronicles 24:20 NKJV)

We **cannot** transgress God's laws and prosper. It won't work, even though we live under grace.

As Paul writes in Romans 3:31, the Law is not made void through faith. Rather we establish it in our hearts, not as any basis of righteousness, but to honour God, who has not changed at all from the Old Testament to the New Testament. Yes, our righteousness is in Christ, but we ignore God's principles at our peril. In other words the God of the Old Testament has not changed, and even though we cannot keep the Law, God does not lower His righteous requirements to accommodate us. On the contrary He expects us to change by the renewing power of the Holy Spirit working in our hearts, while living under grace. It then moves from our heads to our hearts.

Conclusion

God really wants to bless you and to show you His provision as a Father. God has limitless resources, and it is not a big problem for God to prosper you, whether you work with your hands or your brain. I'm reminded of two examples, both very different.

A Christian farmer told me that often he would see the odd cloud coming over his land and dropping just the right amount of rain at the right time, but not doing the same for his neighbour. The right weather is crucial for farmers, and those local to this Christian asked him if he had a hot-line to heaven. Indeed he had. God was prospering him.

I also heard that when NASA first went to the moon they didn't know if the surface was hard or soft. They tried all kinds of test wheels. Then a believer had a dream and God showed him to knit steel like a pan scourer for the wheels. That's what they used. I know believers have received from God complete answers to technical problems in rocket science with words of knowledge. That will certainly prosper your career!

So whether you need more milk from your water buffalos or divine wisdom, Father God can give it to you.

Is there a catch? I don't think so. It's not a game of hide and seek, rather seek and find.

Your giving

"Will a man rob God? Yet you have robbed Me!"
(Malachi 3:8)

If you have not given to God what you owe Him, then the Word of God declares you are under a curse. It has to be put right, so God can open the windows of heaven for you. Too many Christians say they cannot afford to give, so live their lives with cursed finances. Actually you cannot afford to rob God either with the tithe or the free-will offering, and expect blessing.

Your stewardship

It is possible to mismanage money and make bad financial decisions. Some people are good at saving, some just spend, spend, spend, making impulse purchases. Others make no provision for their bills or borrow without thinking through the 'easy terms'. If you know you're bad with money, get some help. Anyone can learn some basic principles and the Bible has lots of advice and instructions about finance.

Curses operating

The most obvious curse is violating God's laws on giving and tithing. I have seen low income believers thrive and prosper and high income people who are constantly short of money.